MY FIRST YEAR

WITH LOVE FROM:

. . . .

WITH LOVE FOR:

. . . .

DATE:

. . . .

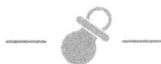

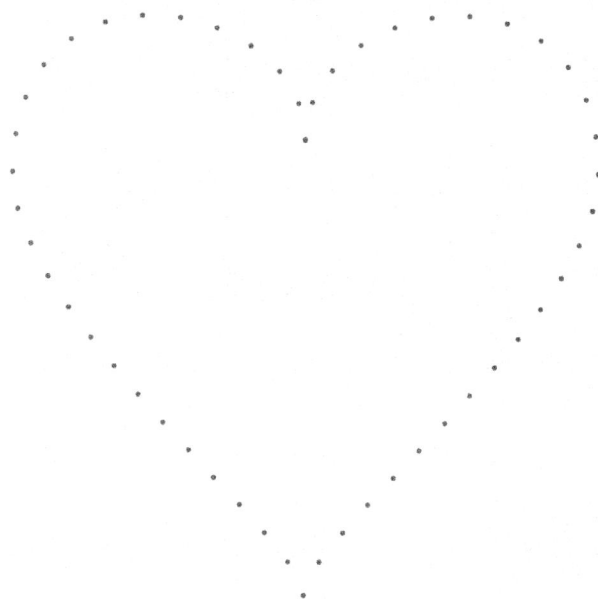

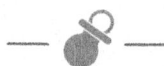

MY FIRST YEAR

MY FIRST YEAR IS FULL OF NEW MOMENTS, EXPERIENCES AND ADVENTURES. FROM THE FIRST WORD TO THE VERY FIRST SHAKY STEPS, I AM EXPERIENCING THE WORLD FOR THE VERY FIRST TIME, DISCOVERING ALL THE THINGS I LIKE (AND POSSIBLY DISLIKE).

THIS BOOK GIVES PARENTS THE OPPORTUNITY TO EXPERIENCE THE FIRST YEAR MORE INTENSIVELY AND HOLD ON TO THOSE PRECIOUS, FUNNY AND BEAUTIFUL MEMORIES FOR YEARS TO COME.

LET'S START OUR MOST EXCITING JOURNEY...

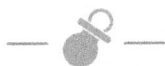

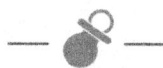

CONTENTS

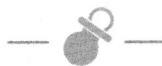

„SO MANY OF
MY SMILES
BEGIN WITH YOU"

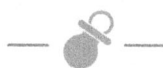

BIRTH

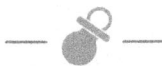

HELLO WORLD – I AM HERE

MY NAME IS:

DATE OF BIRTH:

TIME OF BIRTH:

SIZE:

WEIGHT:

EYE COLOR:

HAIR COLOR:

HEAD CIRCUMFERENCE:

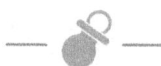

MY FIRST PHOTO:

DATE:

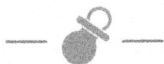

MOMMY'S & DADDY'S FIRST IMPRESSION OF ME IN ONE WORD:

MOMMY

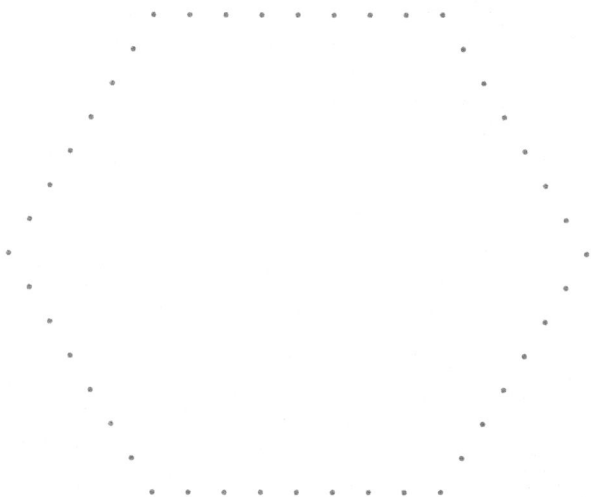

DADDY

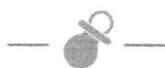

THIS IS HOW MOMMY REALIZED I WANTED TO GET OUT INTO THE WORLD:

THIS IS HOW MY BIRTH WENT:

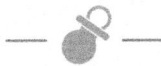

I WAS BORN HERE:

I SMELL LIKE:

MY FIRST SCREAM WAS:

- ○ COMPETING WITH THE SOUND OF A STARTING AIRCRAFT
- ○ THE MOST BEAUTIFUL SOUND IN THE WORLD
- ○ MAGICAL
- ○ PURE HAPPINESS
- ○ SHORT & SWEET
- ○ I HAVE A LONG BREATH
- ○ NONE OF THE ABOVE - IT WAS:

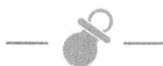

THIS IS HOW OUR FIRST DAY WENT:

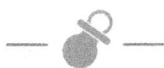

AND OUR FIRST NIGHT WAS LIKE THIS:

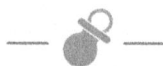

MY FIRST PHOTO WITH MOMMY:

DATE:

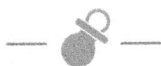

MY FIRST PHOTO WITH DADDY:

DATE:

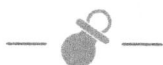

WHAT MOMMY FEELS LIKE WHEN SHE LOOKS AT ME:

AND THIS IS WHAT DADDY THINKS:

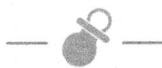

OUR FIRST PHOTO AS A FAMILY:

DATE:

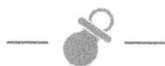

MY FIRST VISITORS WERE:

MESSAGES & WISHES FROM MY VISITORS:

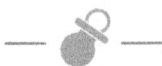

MESSAGES & WISHES FROM MY VISITORS:

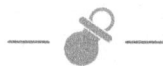

PHOTO OF ME & MY GRANDPARENTS:

DATE:

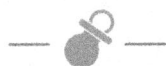

YAY - WE ARE FINALLY GOING HOME AND MY PARENTS ARE LOOKING FORWARD TO:

DATE:

MY NURSERY WAS LOVINGLY DECORATED WITH:

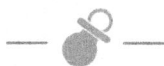

THAT'S ME AT HOME:

PHOTO

DATE:

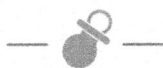

„YOU ARE
MY DEFINITION
OF PERFECT"

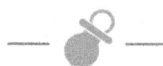

MONTH 1-12

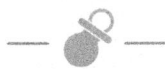

TODAY I AM

1 MONTH

OLD

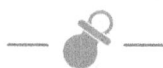

PHOTO

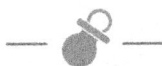

I AM GROWING AND FLOURISHING:

SIZE:

WEIGHT:

HEAD CIRCUMFERENCE:

CLOTHING SIZE:

THIS IS HOW MY FIRST MONTH WAS:

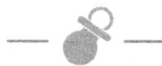

THE MOST BEAUTIFUL MOMENTS:

AND THE BIGGEST CHALLENGES:

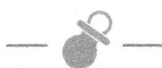

NOTES ON THE PAST MONTH:

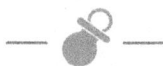

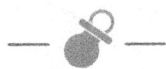

NOW I AM

2 MONTHS

OLD

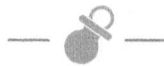

PHOTO

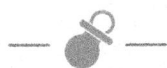

I AM GROWING AND FLOURISHING:

SIZE:

WEIGHT:

HEAD CIRCUMFERENCE:

CLOTHING SIZE:

THIS IS HOW MY SECOND MONTH WAS:

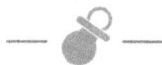

THE MOST BEAUTIFUL MOMENTS:

AND THE BIGGEST CHALLENGES:

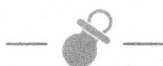

NOTES ON THE PAST MONTH:

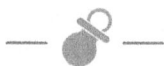

I AM NOW

3 MONTHS

OLD

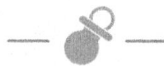

PHOTO

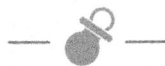

I AM GROWING AND FLOURISHING:

SIZE:

WEIGHT:

HEAD CIRCUMFERENCE:

CLOTHING SIZE:

THIS IS HOW MY THIRD MONTH WAS:

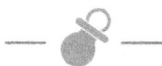

THE MOST BEAUTIFUL MOMENTS:

AND THE BIGGEST CHALLENGES:

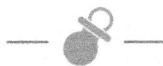

NOTES ON THE PAST MONTH:

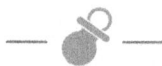

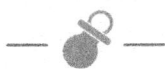

I AM ALREADY

4 MONTHS

OLD

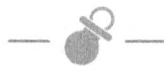

PHOTO

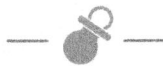

I AM GROWING AND FLOURISHING:

SIZE:

WEIGHT:

HEAD CIRCUMFERENCE:

CLOTHING SIZE:

THIS IS HOW MY FOURTH MONTH WAS:

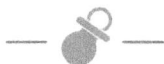

THE MOST BEAUTIFUL MOMENTS:

AND THE BIGGEST CHALLENGES:

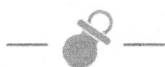

NOTES ON THE PAST MONTH:

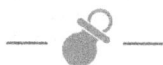

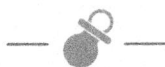

TODAY I AM

5 MONTHS

OLD

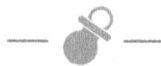

PHOTO

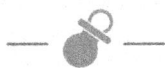

I AM GROWING AND FLOURISHING:

SIZE:

WEIGHT:

HEAD CIRCUMFERENCE:

CLOTHING SIZE:

THIS IS HOW MY FIFTH MONTH WAS:

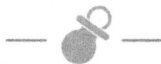

THE MOST BEAUTIFUL MOMENTS:

AND THE BIGGEST CHALLENGES:

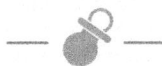

NOTES ON THE PAST MONTH:

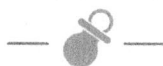

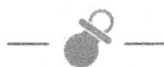

NOW I AM

6 MONTHS

OLD

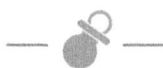

PHOTO

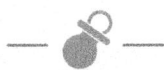

I AM GROWING AND FLOURISHING:

SIZE:

WEIGHT:

HEAD CIRCUMFERENCE:

CLOTHING SIZE:

THIS IS HOW MY SIXTH MONTH WAS:

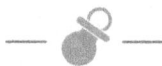

THE MOST BEAUTIFUL MOMENTS:

AND THE BIGGEST CHALLENGES:

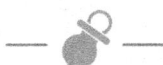

NOTES ON THE PAST MONTH:

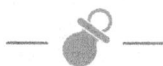

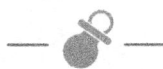

BY NOW I AM ALREADY

7 MONTHS

OLD

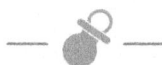

PHOTO

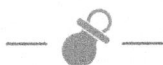

I AM GROWING AND FLOURISHING:

SIZE:

WEIGHT:

HEAD CIRCUMFERENCE:

CLOTHING SIZE:

THIS IS HOW MY SEVENTH MONTH WAS:

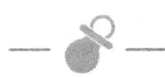

THE MOST BEAUTIFUL MOMENTS:

AND THE BIGGEST CHALLENGES:

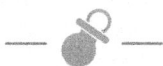

NOTES ON THE PAST MONTH:

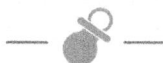

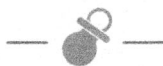

TODAY I AM

8 MONTHS

OLD

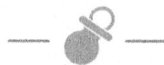

PHOTO

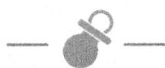

I AM GROWING AND FLOURISHING:

SIZE:

WEIGHT:

HEAD CIRCUMFERENCE:

CLOTHING SIZE:

THIS IS HOW MY EIGHTH MONTH WAS:

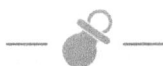

THE MOST BEAUTIFUL MOMENTS:

AND THE BIGGEST CHALLENGES:

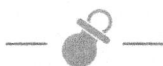

NOTES ON THE PAST MONTH:

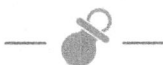

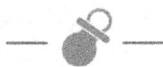

I AM ALREADY

9 MONTHS

OLD

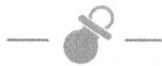

PHOTO

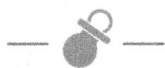

I AM GROWING AND FLOURISHING:

SIZE:

WEIGHT:

HEAD CIRCUMFERENCE:

CLOTHING SIZE:

THIS IS HOW MY NINTH MONTH WAS:

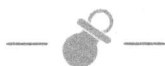

THE MOST BEAUTIFUL MOMENTS:

AND THE BIGGEST CHALLENGES:

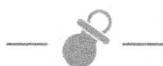

NOTES ON THE PAST MONTH:

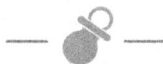

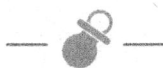

I AM NOW

10 MONTHS

OLD

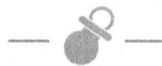

PHOTO

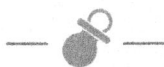

I AM GROWING AND FLOURISHING:

SIZE:

WEIGHT:

HEAD CIRCUMFERENCE:

CLOTHING SIZE:

THIS IS HOW MY TENTH MONTH WAS:

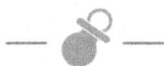

THE MOST BEAUTIFUL MOMENTS:

AND THE BIGGEST CHALLENGES:

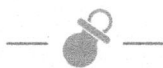

NOTES ON THE PAST MONTH:

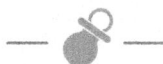

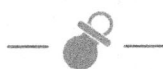

TODAY I AM

11 MONTHS

OLD

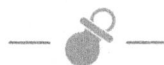

PHOTO

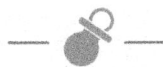

I AM GROWING AND FLOURISHING:

SIZE:

WEIGHT:

HEAD CIRCUMFERENCE:

CLOTHING SIZE:

THIS IS HOW MY ELEVENTH MONTH WAS:

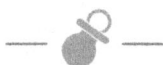

THE MOST BEAUTIFUL MOMENTS:

AND THE BIGGEST CHALLENGES:

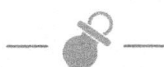

NOTES ON THE PAST MONTH:

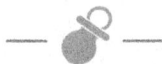

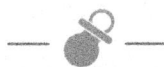

HAPPY BIRTHDAY!

12 MONTHS

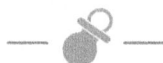

PHOTO

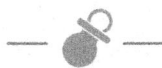

LIST OF MY BIRTHDAY GUESTS:

I RECEIVED THESE WONDERFUL GIFTS:

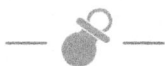

THIS IS HOW WE CELEBRATED;

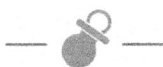

I AM GROWING AND FLOURISHING:

SIZE:

WEIGHT:

HEAD CIRCUMFERENCE:

CLOTHING SIZE:

THIS IS HOW MY TWELFTH MONTH WAS:

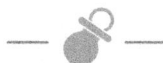

THE MOST BEAUTIFUL MOMENTS:

AND THE BIGGEST CHALLENGES:

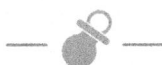

NOTES ON THE PAST MONTH:

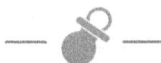

THE MOST BEAUTIFUL MOMENTS OF MY FIRST YEAR:

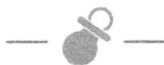

I SOMETIMES DROVE MY PARENTS CRAZY WITH THIS:

MY PARENTS WERE ESPECIALLY PROUD OF:

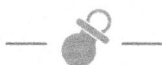

„YOU ARE MY FAVORITE REASON TO LOSE SLEEP"

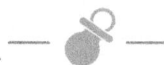

FIRSTS
&
FAVORITES

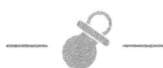

I SMILED FOR THE FIRST TIME TODAY:

PHOTO

DATE:

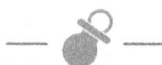

MY FIRST HANDPRINT & FOOTPRINT

DATE:

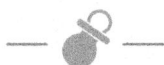

OUR FIRST TRIP LED US HERE & THIS IS WHAT WE DID:

DATE:

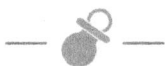

MY FIRST BATH:

PHOTO

DATE:

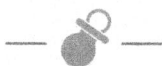

I ROLLED OVER FOR THE FIRST TIME TODAY:

DATE:

I SAID „MOMMY" FOR THE FIRST TIME TODAY:

DATE:

I SAID „DADDY" FOR THE FIRST TIME TODAY:

DATE:

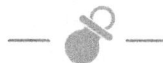

MY FIRST WORD

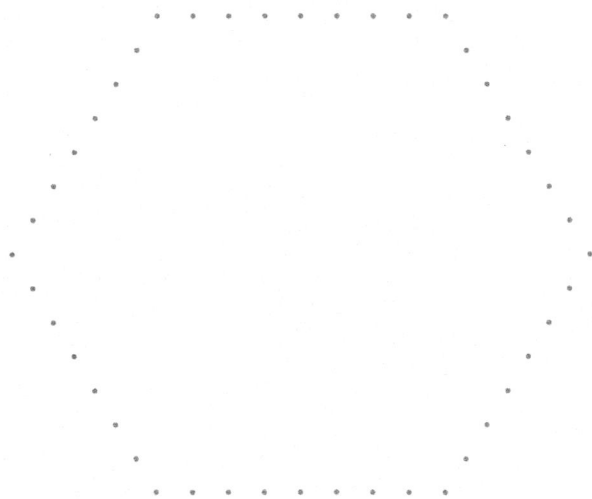

DATE:

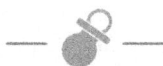

I CAN SIT UP ALL BY MYSELF:

PHOTO

DATE:

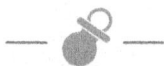

AND NOW I CAN EVEN STAND UP:

PHOTO

DATE:

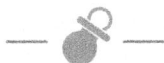

TODAY I ATE SOLID FOOD FOR THE FIRST TIME AND I THOUGHT IT WAS:

DATE:

I SLEPT THROUGH THE ENTIRE NIGHT FOR THE FIRST TIME TODAY:

DATE:

MY FIRST TOOTH APPEARED AND THIS IS HOW IT MADE ME FEEL:

DATE:

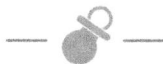

I TOOK MY FIRST STEPS TODAY:

PHOTO

DATE:

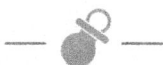

MY MOST BELOVED CUDDLY TOY:

MY FAVORITE FOOD:

THIS IS WHAT I LIKE TO DRINK THE MOST:

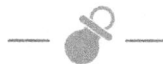

MY NUMBER ONE BOOK:

MY FAVORITE WORD:

WHAT I LOVE DOING THE MOST:

MY DEAREST ANIMAL:

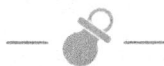

MY FAVORITE SONG:

THE LYRICS OF MY FINEST LULLABY:

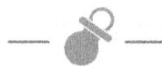

MY DEAREST PLAYMATES:

MY TOY OF CHOICE:

MY NUMBER ONE COLOR:

MY FAVORITE PLACES:

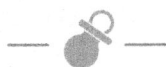

SPACE FOR MEMORIES, STORIES & WISHES:

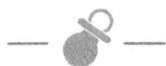

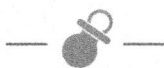

ON OUR OWN BEHALF

FIRST OF ALL, WE WOULD LIKE TO SAY A HEARTFELT THANK YOU, FOR YOUR TRUST IN OUR PRODUCT. IF YOU LIKED THIS BOOK AND YOU KEEP GOING THROUGH IT WITH A SMILE ON YOUR FACE, THEN WE HAVE ACHIEVED OUR MOST IMPORTANT GOAL. WE PUT A LOT OF LOVE INTO OUR BOOKS AND WOULD BE REALLY HAPPY IF YOU CHOOSE TO GIVE US A REVIEW.

FEEL FREE TO CHECK OUT OUR OTHER KUOSIA PRODUCTS, YOU MIGHT EVEN FIND SOME OTHER BOOKS YOU LIKE.

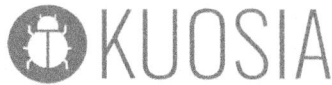

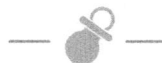

Made in the USA
Coppell, TX
01 March 2023